Assault on
Binge Eating Disorder

By

Aaron Capp

This book was written to identify, understand and cope with binge eating disorder.

To

Diana

This book would not have been written without her

NOTICE: You Do NOT Have the
Right to Reprint This Book

Introduction

I have a good friend name Jill; it is hard not to be a friend of hers for she is such a warm and friendly person. Although I have notice is the past, she seems to gain weight and then go on a crush diet. Well not a diet, she simply doesn't eat for days.

She appears to lose and gain back weight more often and has become almost paranoid about gaining weight. When I talk to her about starving herself, she gets offensive. So I don't bring it up very often.

She seems to be unhappy at times. I'm a true friend and would like to help her. I don't think her actions are normal.

1

What is Bing Eating Disorder?

Binge eating is as much an eating disorder as anorexia or bulimia. Although anorexics and bulimics are physically capable of being distinguished, binge eaters disguise themselves as normal weight, or overweight individuals.

It is estimated that binge eating disorder is actually more common and frequent than anorexia or bulimia.

The Mayo Clinic defines binge eating disorder (BED) as a "serious eating disorder in which you frequently consume unusually large amounts of food".

Now it is true the most people over eat occasionally such as having second or even third helpings of a holiday meal, but this is not the case of a person having binge eating disorder.

Assault On Binge Eating Disorder

In the United States binge eating disorder is the most common eating disorder, but is still not classified as a distinct psychiatrics condition, a condition that would cause mental illness or instability.

But if you have BED self-help treatment will help you. Binge eating disorder usually leads to obesity although it can occur in normal weight individuals.

2

What are the characteristics of Binge Eating Disorder?

One can think that Binge Eating is a form of over eating at its worst. As by definition it can affect all ages, both men or women, or race, although it is most common eating disorder it is one of the least known.

Here some characteristics of Binge Eating Disorder:

1. Binge episode – a person will overeat much faster than normal in a short period of time (just a couple of hours) and at times lose complete control. They eat until uncomfortably full or even sick. These episodes are often and the person may or may not be hungry.

Gain weight excessively or sudden onset of obesity will cause mental as well as physical problems.

2. Binges more than twice a week for as long as six months, and then may feel disgusted with themselves, depressed, bored or guilty about their eating habit. Binge eaters have a different relationship with food. Binge eaters believe they have no control in what or how much they can eat especially when they begin eating.

3. It is not uncommon to find binge eaters overweight and unhappy about themselves. A BED person is usually overweight, but not always, because of the high calories they consume, this at times causes stress the will result in eating even more.

It is important to realize the extra fat a binge eater carries can cause heart disease, diabetes, and other medical conditions.

4. Binge eaters will search for outside sources to cure their disorder such as dieting, hoping to regulate the amount of food they take in. But what happens is they go from one diet to another hoping to find the perfect solution only to relapse into binging between diets.

The binger is constantly preoccupied with diets and food talking about it constantly even over meals, but avoids social situations because of their circumstance in most cases of being fat.

They truly believe that they would be happy if they were thin. It is truly unclear whether dieting and binge eating are related, even when they binge after dieting. It is not usually the binger considers dieting as simply skipping meals or not eating enough during meal time or simply avoiding certain kinds of food.

Dieting also lowers your metabolism causing the body to reduce the process of burning fat.

Of course this is extremely unhealthy diets.

5. Another characteristic of a person with binge eating disorder is they will try to stay busy to avoid eating. The belief here is if you are idle you will way to tried to change your weight or body shape, and this will also lose more self-esteem because of failed begin eating, because they have nothing to do.

When they do eat their lunch or dinner with friends or family they will eat low calorie items, but in private they eat high calorie food such as candy, cakes, cookies, desserts and almost any sugary food, and of course will lie about what they have eaten.

6. As touch on before a person that has binge eating disorder eats much more quickly during these binge period that during normal eating period. At this point a person is truly a food addict.

This eating larger and larger amount of food is a true characteristic of a binge eater. During this time of heavy eating the person has complete lack of control. After this period the person will feel guilty, begin skipping meals such as breakfast, avoid certain high calorie content foods, and buy most foods that are used for diets.

7. At this point the binger will feel embarrassed, disgusted, ashamed, depressed, guilty or even angry with themselves after a binge eating period. Researchers have found as many as half of the people with this disorder are depressed or have been depressed in their past.

Because of this it is difficult to determine whether depression causes binge eating disorder or whether in fact the disorder causes depression. Other research studies suggest people who have binge eating disorder may have a problem handing some of their emotions. Many bingers who have been interviewed say that they have a hard time not binge eating when emotions such as stress, anger, being bored, and worry embroil them.

Reviewing some of the symptoms of binge eating disorder may give you an idea as to whether you have or have not this serious problem.

But you must keep in mind not all binge eaters act in the same way so that not all symptoms may apply.

Remember that bingeing is totally different than overeating, that we all do from time to time. It is true that we occasional overdo it, such as special occasions or holiday meals. Were as a person with binge eating disorder has little control over what, when and how much food they put into their bodies.

The Clinical Guidelines on the Identification, Evaluation, and Treatment of Overweight and Obesity in Adults, published in 1998 by the National Heart, Lung, and Blood Institute, define overweight as a body mass index (BMI) of 25 to 29.9 and obesity as a BMI of 30 or more. BMI is calculated by dividing weight (in kilograms) by height (in meters) squared.

3

Self Help & Treatment for Binging

If you have come to the conclusion that you are a binge eater and now want change your life. So where do you go from here. This is a time where things can be a little scary. You are going into unfamiliar territory. You know that you want to get rid of this disorder, but you might be thinking what I will be like without it.

You will be changing the way you live. Will you be better or worse? These thoughts can make any one nervous. Maybe you turned to food to solve your problems for so long you don't know what to do if that crutch is gone. You know you do not want to eat yourself to death, but you eat because you have been doing it so long, you don't know any other way.

I believe Jill has this disorder and if you believe you have it too you can solve this problem through a manta affirmation. I will show you how this is done.

It is now time to look at your lifestyle since you realize that you have a binge eating disorder problem. You must develop simple practical steps that will stop cold this disorder.

Let me give you a little background.

It is now the time to change your feelings through mantas using affirmations. It is through your mantra you will be able to change. People can be scared because they believe they are entering unknown territory.

But it will be different with you, because you will create a plan by simply making a list of "power words (affirmations)" and using your mantra you will know exactly where you are going. Going down the road to a new and better life, you planned out your destination by yourself. The risk many people feel are not your feelings, you know what future is in store for you, because you are building your own future.

With your mantra you created positive thoughts your mind will absorb. Through your affirmations you will become a healthier person. You will become a better person, the old you will disappear. The person you will become will begin to like itself.

The double life you led, hiding your binging, will disappear. You will know longer worry about when you will binge next. You will even begin to have a normal relationship with food. What is more important you will finally be happy about your life, something you probably have dreamed about for a long time?

So when bad thoughts start turning into good thoughts, you will notice the change isn't all that scary. As a matter of fact, you will probably get excited rather than scared. You will reach a point when you can hardly wait for the next part of your life to unfold.

But the engine that drives you, making you go forward is your motivation. You have decided you want to get rid of binge eating disorder. You have set out a plan. You have derived the affirmation mantras to change your life.

It will be the motivation that drives you to your destination after you make decision to move forward. It is truly the fuel that keeps the motor driving you to your final destination. It is positive change that creates positive motivation.

A person taking positive actions to become a better person will begin to like him/herself.

When you determine you going to kick out the habit of binge eating disorder, it is the positive motivation that will drive you and anyone else to their final goal. To be more exact it is motivation that will raise the bar to hurl you in the right direction.

As that positive change starts in your life through your motivation you will want more. It will continuously push you forward. Obstacle you had thought were impossible to overcome will fade away in front of you. It is important that your grasp this concept. With positive motivation, hard work, and dedication you will prevail.

What the most important aspect to the journey to recovery is *your commitment*. Without total commitment your journey will end before it really starts.

Throw all the junk food you eat in the trash. I know this will be hard, but if you are committed, you must do this.

4

Beginning of the End of BED

Humans are creatures of habit; it can become obvious as to the cause of the problem. And because we are creatures of habit, we build on to our past habits. Because of habits a good life can change you forever.

A few notes before we start meditation:

Wikipedia defines meditation as "any of a family of practices in which practitioners train their minds or self-induce a mode of consciousness to realize benefit.

Meditation is generally an inwardly oriented, personal practice, which individuals can do by themselves. Meditation may involve invoking or cultivating a feeling or internal state, such as compassion, or attending to a specific focal point.

The type of meditation you will be using is a mantra with an affirmation.

The mind is truly lazy and doesn't want to stay focused on one thing. It doesn't want to concentrate and as you focus on one thought other thoughts will appear.

It is important to push those thoughts away and get back to your single thought. Don't give up; this is the normal process of the mind. Every time a random thought appears, push it aside and get back to your focused thought.

Something you might not know is the mind doesn't recognize a negative word. So if you don't want to think, let's say cars. You wouldn't want to say "Don't think about cars." The mind will drop don't and began thinking about cars.

So you don't want to think in the negative. The key to removing binge eating disorder from your life is to add positive affirmations to your meditation.

How long will it take? Good question. Positive affirmations you feel good about saying will change you quickly. Others that you dislike are getting resistance which is good don't give up on them, these will solve your deep rooted problems.

Here are some positive affirmations you can use:

- Every Cell in my body vibrates with energy and health

- Loving me heals my life. I nourish my mind, body and soul

- My body heals quickly and easily

- I am the perfect weight for me

- I choose to make positive healthy choices for myself

- I choose to exercise regularly

The key to removing binge eating disorder from your life is to add positive affirmations to your meditation.

These are some ideas, but you can make up your own positive affirmations to fit your situation.

At first you will send most of your time learning to relax, with little on meditation. So you might want to start with five to ten minutes a day in the beginning.

So let's start, right now, read the steps, put the book down and begin:

Step 1: First the position, what is most comfortable to you: just sitting in a chair legs slightly apart, maybe cross legged on the floor on a cushion, or you might want to be in a yoga style position on the floor with the full lotus position, it's up to you. The major element is for you to be *comfortable*.

Step 2: Now you need to sit straight but also be comfortable (this might be hard, but try doing it). Try having the weight of your head be directly on your spinal column. Sometimes it helps if you pull in your chin a little. If you are sitting on the floor let the small of your back to be slightly arched. But remember do not get into any gyrations that you are not comfortable in.

Step 3: Place your tongue against the roof of your mouth. Closing your mouth, begin breathing through you nose.

Step 4: At this point you need to become aware. Close your eyes and begin to focus.

First, what is your body touching such as the chair you're sitting in or the cushion if you're on the floor? What do you feel touching it? What sensations do you feel when your body is touching itself. How does it feel, your legs cross on the floor, or maybe your arms cross as you sit down. Become aware of the places that your body is in contact with, whether it's part of the body or outside the body.

Second, Now note how your body is place in its surroundings, how much space is it taking up. Can you feel the boundaries between you and the space around you?

Step 5: Now it's time to sense your body with your eyes still close. How is your breathing? Is it fast or slow? Is it deep or shallow? Where is your breath seated? Is it down low below your stomach? Is it in the middle of your stomach? Is it high in your chest?

Now try moving your breath from one area to another. Try this, it might be hard at first, breathe into your upper chest, then into your stomach, than drop to below your stomach in your belly with practice you can do it, and be proud of it.

With the breathing in the lower stomach you will notice that the upper chest and the stomach are almost quiet, not moving. This known as the "dropped breath" and is believed to be the most relaxing stance to meditate from. As I said before, don't worry it will come to you with practice.

Step 6: Now as you relaxed, it is time to say your positive affirmation mantra. Say it over and over again in your mind. It is not uncommon, again especially when you first start, that your mind will stray, thinking of other thoughts.

Slowly pull it back to your mantra, and start again repeating your special mantra. Don't force it; let it find its own speed or rhythm. It will come as you continuously repeat it. If you are alone begin to speak it out loud, let your voice fill you and let it relax you more.

Be unyielding about the time you spend each day. It is good if you can pick a certain place and time each day for your meditation. You are getting a rid of an eating disorder, this is important; it will change your life, in many ways if you stick to it.

A problem you can handle with this book.

.It's time to change your lifestyle

Turn over a new leaf, be committed...

One of the best ways to clear your mine before or even after your meditation sessions is simply taking a walk. So whenever possible take a long walk in nature. Enjoy the day and what GOD has given us. Feel the wind and watch the trees as they sway. Listen to birds chirping back and forth.

Take in a deep breath and smell the fresh air. A long an enjoyable walk is one of the best things to toss away your troubles and to relax you. What had seen major before the walk will be minor obstacles that you now can handle.

As your mind and body become stronger in resisting the disorder, you will become stronger, and feel better about yourself, you will start loving yourself.

So in conclusion – don't be afraid to stop binge eating and begin your new life.